To my mother, Jodi Morell. She has supported me throughout my life to the best of her ability, and for that, I am grateful.

Tia

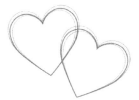

OBSESSED WITH MINDFUL EATING
A HEART-CENTERED APPROACH TO NUTRITION

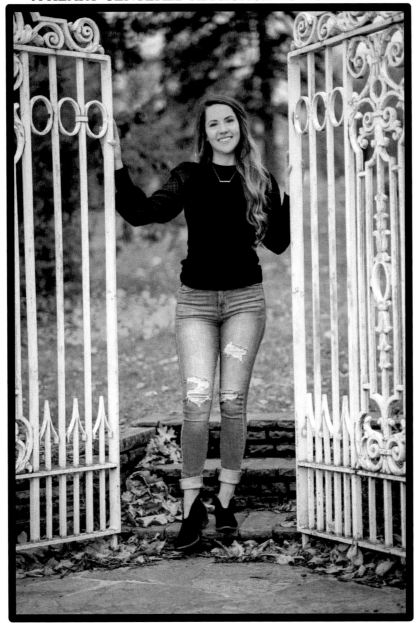

By Tia Morell

Dear Reader,

I am obsessed with Tia Morell.

This statement may seem dramatic, but honestly, she inspires me to do better and be better. I have had the privilege of inhabiting the space that is "Tia" for almost two years. During this time, I have witnessed an evolution of self-discovery that is remarkable. Her instinct to grow isn't hindered by a backdrop of anxiety or fear. Instead, she properly addresses mind-blocks, "does the work," and discovers new paths that align with her mission to empower and educate the women around her.

Let's rewind. Bear with me as I paint the picture of a young woman grappling with self-confidence, self-awareness, and a sprinkling of self-doubt. Tia was caged by her body, caught in a downward spiral, believing that being skinny meant she was living her dream life. However, when she achieved her goal, a feeling of emptiness lingered.

I met Tia long after she struggled with body image. I met her when she radiated grace in her journey. It was hard to miss, as she humbly professed that she loved herself just as she was. She embraced the messy. She flaunted her flaws. And she had more confidence in herself than ever before. Tia is a Unicorn who imparts her no-nonsense approach to food and helps women untangle their complicated relationships with eating. She teaches women if they love themselves, the rest will follow.

While working together in coaching and podcasting, she has become my friend. I have become a student of her philosophy on compassion. Fortunately, the time I spend with her is laden with truth bombs. This book shares this wisdom with you. So, sit at the scrumptious table of Tia, and devour her lessons. This book you are about to read is your access to her undeniable teachings presented with her brand of grace.

I have no doubt that you will refer to this primer on Mindful Eating regularly. I know you will become as obsessed with Tia as I am.

Julie Lokun, JD
Autor of *HustleSmart: The Ultimate Guide for New Entrepreneurs*

Table of Contents

CHAPTER 1 A HEART-CENTERED APPROACH TO NUTRITION 1

    PRE-ASSESSMENT 5

CHAPTER 2 WHAT IS MINDFUL EATING? 7

    BEING HEART-CENTERED 8

    SIMILAR EATING PHILOSOPHIES 9

    LISTENING TO YOUR BODY 10

    INFLUENCES 11

    YOU ARE IN CONTROL 12

CHAPTER 3 PREPARING YOUR MINDSET 15

    STEP ONE: REJECT DIET CULTURE 15

    STEP 2: STOP COMPARING YOURSELF TO OTHERS 16

CHAPTER 4 THE BENEFITS OF MINDFUL EATING 21

    FOOD FOR THOUGHT 21

    GAINING CONTROL 22

    BALANCE 24

CHAPTER 5 HOW TO EAT MINDFULLY 27

    START WITH SMALL CHANGES 27

    TRY IT OUT! 28

    SLOW DOWN! 28

    REMEMBER THESE TIPS: 31

    KEEP A JOURNAL 35

CHAPTER 6 EATING WHOLE FOODS 37

    THE IMPORTANCE OF WHOLE FOODS 37

    THE VIBRATIONAL ENERGY OF FOOD 37

    FIBER 39

    ORGANIC? YES OR NO? 41

    POWER FOODS 42

CHAPTER 7 PRIMARY FOODS 45

    PRIMARY FOODS 45

CHAPTER 8 EATING FOR HAPPINESS 51

    FOOD AND MOOD 51

CHAPTER 9 TREATING YOURSELF WITH KINDNESS AND COMPASSION 57

LOVE YOURSELF 57

SELF-CARE 58

STAY HYDRATED 61

GET OUTSIDE... 62

EXERCISE 64

SLEEP... 65

FIND WHAT WORKS FOR YOU 67

CHAPTER 10 THE IMPORTANCE OF KINDNESS..................................... 69

BE KIND AND BRAVE 69

POSITIVE AFFIRMATIONS: 70

BEING INTENTIONAL 72

CHAPTER 11 WRAP-UP 75

POST ASSESSMENT 77

CHAPTER 12 IN THE KITCHEN 81

Green Smoothie 81

Veggie Pasta Salad... 82

Pasta and Veggies 83

"Stuffed' Recipe 84

Great for stuffing mushrooms, bell peppers, jalapenos, tomatoes, and more! 84

Zucchini Lasagna 85

Whole Meal Salad Outline.. 87

Whole Meal Template 88

CHAPTER 13 RESOURCES 89

CHAPTER 1
A HEART-CENTERED APPROACH TO NUTRITION

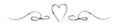

"It is the health that is real wealth and not pieces of gold and silver."- Mahatma Gandhi

It is important to have a heart-centered approach when taking responsibility for your health.

Dear Reader,
My family has discussed weight standards and diet culture for as long as I can remember. Since I was considered a chubby child, I became obsessed with body image and weight at a young age.

I was also labeled with a learning disability in Elementary School and was separated from my classmates to participate in individual instruction. This heightened my awareness that I was different from my peers. I started comparing myself not just physically but intellectually. This led to severe anxiety and increasing issues with body image.

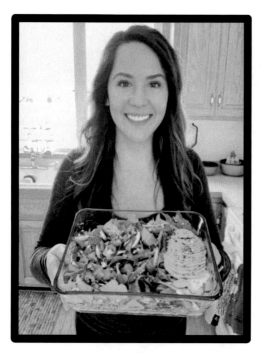

Although my family was close and supportive, there was a lack of education on mental health, so self-esteem issues were not discussed or dealt with. I learned to shove my feelings deep inside. Then I was encouraged to fit into my surroundings the best that I could. Only in hindsight can I see that anxiety was driving both my struggle with digestive issues and my hatred of school.

Once I hit middle school, I grew out of my baby weight, but poor body image continued to plague me. I remained obsessed with keeping my weight down and fitting in. I wouldn't do anything that made me stand out.

By the time I hit high school, I was obsessed with weighing myself. This led to my first diet. I replaced some meals with prepackaged diet products, and I skipped others. I loved the results I saw on the scale. Hence, my yo-yo dieting craze began. My self-worth was tied to the number on the scale and fitting in with my peers. I was a follower, not a leader, and I thought I had found the way to fit in.

In college, I felt lost. I didn't know who I was or what I wanted out of life. I gained weight in the first two years and wanted to lose it as quickly as possible. I tried every quick fix I found on Pinterest, in magazines, and through word of mouth. I was reintroduced to meal skipping, calorie counting, and the number on the scale. I once again developed an unhealthy obsession with my weight. I was doing things not because I wanted to but because I felt I had to. Life felt meaningless. I partied a lot and had an all-or-nothing mentality about food. I would restrict myself in unhealthy ways during the week and binge eat and drink on the weekends. I was miserable most of the time, and depression hit me hard. I wasn't looking forward to the future. I didn't even want to acknowledge or walk at graduation.

I had no choice but to be honest with myself and my parents about my internal battles. My doctor prescribed medication for anxiety, depression, and sleeping. However, I continued to live the same lifestyle and engaged in the poor eating habits I developed in college.

Six months after graduation, I was in a four-wheeler accident that left me bedridden for about one month and in a wheelchair for almost four months. This was the wake-up call I needed to change. I promised myself I would focus on health and wellness once I could walk again. Unfortunately, I tried another fad diet to lose weight and again found myself skipping meals.

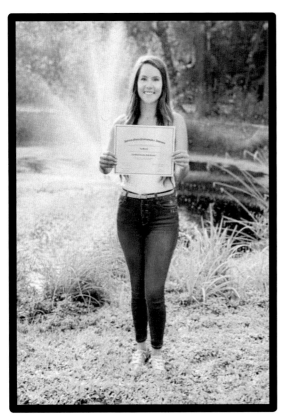

I have spent most of my life convinced I wasn't skinny enough. I thought if I hit that magic number on the scale, I would finally be happy, and life would be great. The day I hit my goal weight, I looked in the mirror and didn't recognize who I saw. I was still unhappy, anxious, and depressed. That's when I realized my lifestyle, diet, and environment worked against me, not for me.

Fear of change and being uncomfortable with putting my authentic self first paralyzed me. It took me over a year and a half to take the leap and change my environment. This was the springboard that launched my healthier lifestyle and the diet changes I desired. I spent the time I needed on me, myself, and I. As my wise mother often reminds me, these are the three most important people in my life.

With conscious effort, I figured out who I was at my core and installed habits that aligned with my values. I saw changes in my mental, emotional, and physical health that I never thought possible. I am grateful to have experienced firsthand the impacts that lifestyle, diet, and environment have on overall health.

This newfound knowledge inspired me to earn my Holistic Nutritionist certification and become certified with The Institute for Integrative Nutrition. I now view health in a new light and love encouraging others who are struggling.

I hope that my story helps others. Now, instead of being obsessed with the number on the scale, I am obsessed with humans on the verge of change.

With Love,
Tia

PRE-ASSESSMENT

Before reading this book grab a piece of paper and complete this assessment.

Self Assesment

Where do you fall with these statements? Where do you want to fall with them? How can you start to implement mindful eating habits into your life?

1. I take the time to notice how hungry I am before I start eating to make the appropriate food choices and control the portion size?

2. I eat my meals while watching TV, scrolling social media, listening to audio, reading emails, text, or making calls?

3. I eat to the point of being uncomfortable? I often want to do 'nothing' after I eat?

4. I eat so quickly I barely taste the food, notice the texture, think about the appearance or appreciate how it got on my plate?

5. I find myself staring into the refrigerator/pantry for reasons other than being hungry?

Self Assessment
Page 2

6. When I notice my attention drifting during meals, I refocus my thoughts back to the eating experience?

7. When I feel hungry my first instinct is to avoid the feeling and distract myself so I don't eat?

8. I always finish my plate, even when I know I am full before all the food is gone?

9. I make food choices based on the quality and quantity of what those around me eat?

10. I accept my body as is at all times without judgment?

CHAPTER 2

WHAT IS MINDFUL EATING?

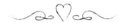

"Your present circumstances don't determine where you can go; they merely determine where you start." -Nido Qubein

Energy flows where focus goes" is a mantra I live by. If we become stuck in a negative loop of hating ourselves, our bodies will respond to that with the same energy caliber. Love is the energy that moves your life forward. By embracing love, compassion, and gratitude, you expand your life beyond what you imagine possible. When you intentionally choose to cultivate a loving energy towards yourself, you start to choose foods that embody this same quality.

I believe in having a **heart-centered** approach to health. I encourage people to eat with full awareness. I tell them not to judge their thoughts, feelings, and emotions that come up while nourishing their body. I advocate being mindful of the process, **engaging in self-love, and being present during every moment.**

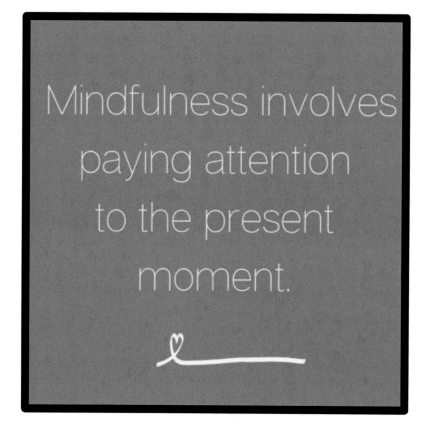

When someone mentions food, where does your mind go? Do you think about changing the way you currently eat? Do you think of the last diet you went on or the next one you plan to try? Do you feel guilt or shame around your current eating habits?

Mindful Eating can help alleviate these negative feelings about food because it is a non-judgemental approach that focuses on sensual awareness of the food instead of calories, carbohydrates, fat, and protein. Mindful Eating puts your full awareness on the eating experience and pays attention to your body's signals to hunger and satiety. The purpose of eating this way is not to lose weight, although many people who adopt this eating style will see the number on the scale go down. Mindful Eating encourages savoring the moment as well as the flavor, texture, and look of food. It enables you to be fully present for the eating experience.

The important things to keep in mind are that mindfulness focuses on appreciating the entire eating experience and choosing what and how much to consume. With a mindful approach, most people eat less, savor the experience, and select foods with desirable health benefits.

SIMILAR EATING PHILOSOPHIES

I am often asked about the differences between Mindful Eating, Intuitive Eating, and Compassionate Eating. Although the three philosophies are compatible, there are differences. Compassionate Eating looks at how what you eat affects the world. Mindful Eating is learning to be present and in the moment. Intuitive Eating is an approach used by nutritionists to teach individuals not to be afraid of food and to listen to their body cues.

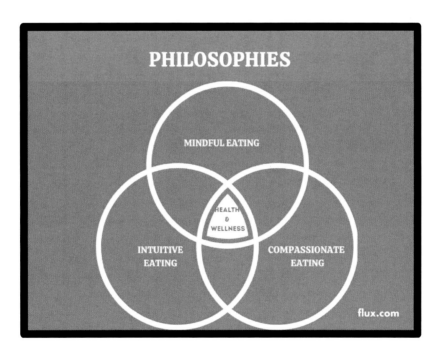

Let's delve deeper into these philosophies.

Intuitive Eating: Incorporates the idea that you are the expert on what your body needs. It involves listening to your body, following your innate hunger and satiety cues, and indulging in what your body craves. Intuitive eating helps you restore the wisdom you were born with when it comes to food. It is a system that nutritionists use to empower individuals with eating disorders.

Compassionate Eating: Incorporates the philosophy that mind, body, spirit, and planet all matter when choosing what food to eat. The following questions must be asked before consuming anything: *Have any animals been harmed to provide my food? Has Mother Earth been adversely affected while providing my food? Have the workers that provided my food been treated fairly?*

Mindful Eating: Incorporates an in-the-moment awareness of food. It is influenced by Buddist thought.

As you can see, the three philosophies overlap, and all three have the same end goal—making choices that are best for you and your health. I will focus on Mindful Eating in this book.

LISTENING TO YOUR BODY

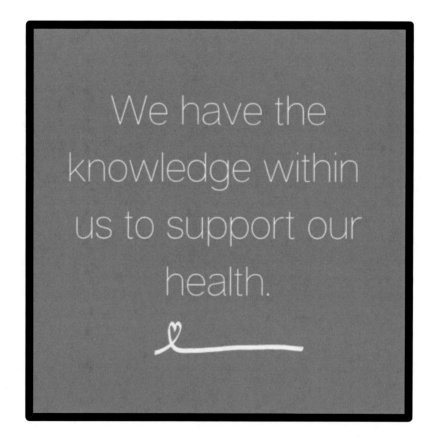

We have the knowledge within us to support our health.

You have the knowledge within you to support your health. Biologically your body knows what it needs to thrive, and when you learn to trust yourself, you will make choices that set you up for success.

I promise you, the benefits of tuning into your body are well worth the challenges.

INFLUENCES

How we grew up; what those around us eat; what schools serve; what advertisements we are exposed to; and what we buy at stores and seek out in restaurants affect us on both a conscious and unconscious level.

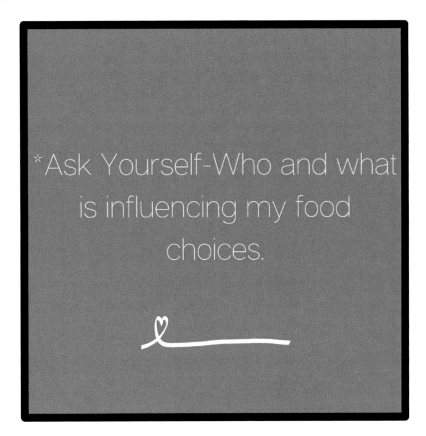

Billions of dollars are spent to influence our food choices. We have become victims of the food industry's bombardment of advertisements and confusing labels. Then we mix in diet culture and indecipherable studies. This massive pile of confusion often leads you to choose harmful foods. It isn't a coincidence or bad luck that chronic diseases are on the rise. You aren't alone if it feels as though you aren't in complete control of your food choices.

The good news is that by learning to be mindful, you can ignore the bad influences and unlock your innate knowledge.

YOU ARE IN CONTROL

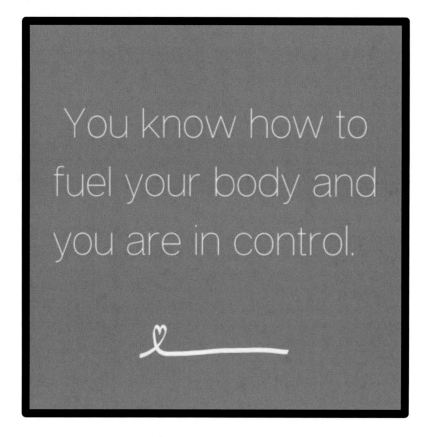

Take control by becoming aware of who and what is influencing your food choices. Then implement small shifts to make changes in your diet and lifestyle that will positively impact your quality of life.

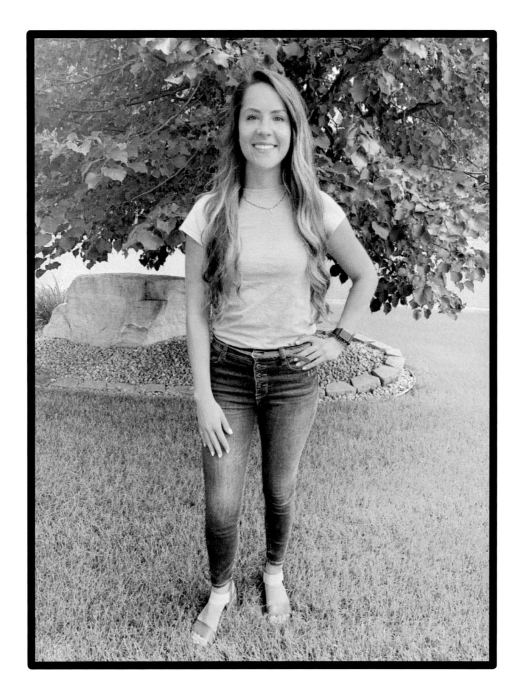

CHAPTER 3

PREPARING YOUR MINDSET

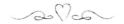

"The mind is everything. What you think you become." – Buddha

Mindset is the most crucial part of having a heart-centered approach to healthy nutrition. The following positive actions will get you started on your journey.

STEP ONE: REJECT DIET CULTURE

Diet culture profits off insecurities. It makes you believe your self-worth is tied to a number on the scale. It encourages obsessiveness about how you look externally compared to others and ignores how you feel internally. It forces you to believe that if you follow that diet, use

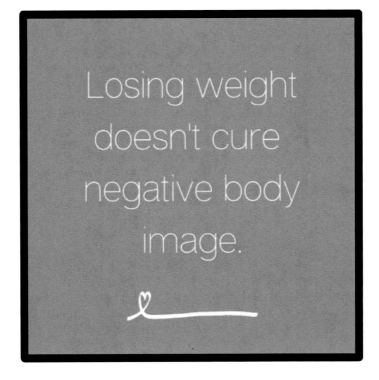

this exercise program, or take "healthy" supplements, you will look like the beautiful photoshopped individuals flashed in your face. And, only then, will your body be loveable. I say enough is enough. We are all born worthy!

STEP 2: STOP COMPARING YOURSELF TO OTHERS

What does healthy look like?

Most people want a straightforward answer, but we are all a different kind of healthy. We aren't going to be the same weight, height, or shape as the person standing beside us. Therefore, healthy looks different for each one of us.

Why should anyone hate themselves because they feel they don't measure up to society's standards? When you look in the mirror and feel a rush of negativity bubble up, recognize this unhealthy mindset.

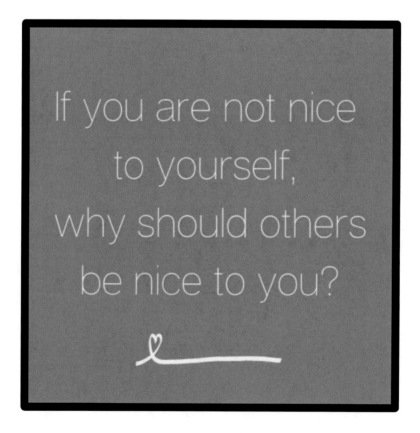

If you start the day wondering why you can't be more like so-and-so, you will find all of the negatives you are looking for. Remember, you **attract what you give off. Are you attracting the things you desire or the things you fear?** Think of self-fulfilling prophecies. This comparison mindset doesn't set you up for success.

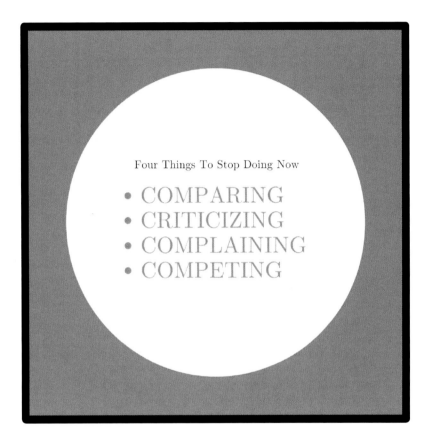

Four Things To Stop Doing Now
- COMPARING
- CRITICIZING
- COMPLAINING
- COMPETING

I often tell my clients, "Turn those negative thoughts around. Don't let them take hold of you."

Just because you have a thought doesn't make it true. Know that you can change your mindset. **You are in control, and** the first thing that you can do is bring awareness to your thoughts.

Start here. Recognize those hurtful words you tell yourself because identifying negative patterns can be liberating.

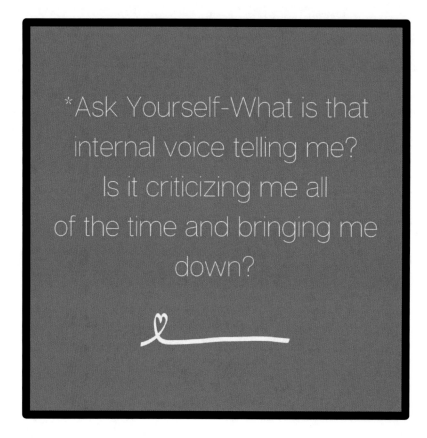

*Ask Yourself-What is that internal voice telling me? Is it criticizing me all of the time and bringing me down?

It is essential to take a look around and be honest with yourself. Who do you surround yourself with? Who are your idols? Who embodies your overall health goals. Whose body do you try to emulate?

The critical thing to realize is that you may be comparing yourself to someone's highlight reel **or social mask.** You don't see the breakdown they just had or their sink full of dirty dishes. You don't know that X, Y, and Z just went wrong in their life. You don't see their belly roll over their jeans when they sit. You see the flattering angles. You see the photoshopped images and get an unrealistic idea of what health is and what health isn't. This is very black and white thinking, and it is an all-or-nothing mindset.
What do healthy people have in common?

They know that comparison is the thief of joy. When comparing yourself to others, you inevitably feel bad about yourself. Life is a journey that you should celebrate right now, and it is too short to deprive yourself of a single moment of joy that comparison steals from you.

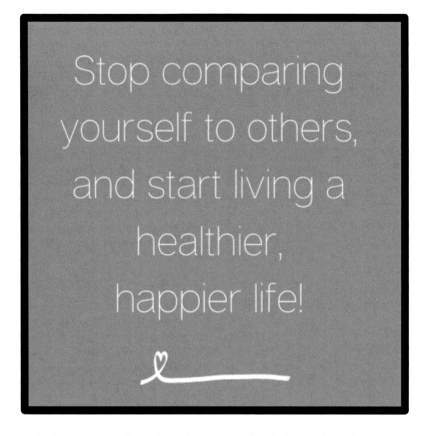

Stop comparing yourself to others, and start living a healthier, happier life!

Remember, catch those nasty thoughts. Stop them in their tracks. The more you practice, the more mindful you will become and the easier it will become to redirect unwelcome ideas.

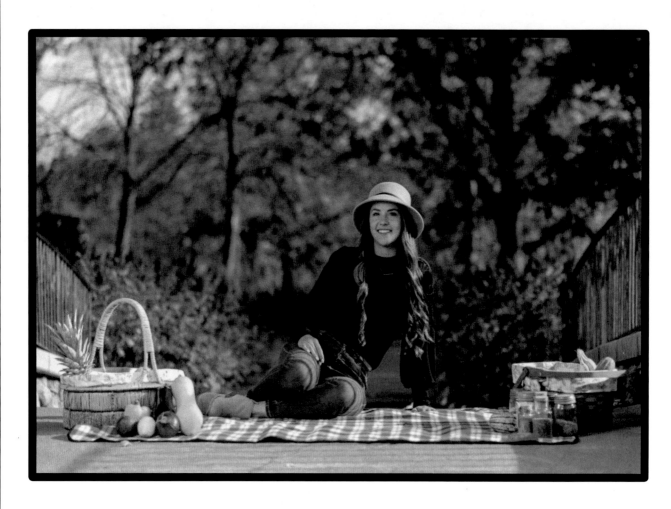

CHAPTER 4

THE BENEFITS OF MINDFUL EATING

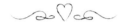

"Healthy citizens are the greatest asset any country can have."- Winston Churchill

I wish I could take back the time I wasted on restricting and depriving my body of food in an attempt to be skinny. Thankfully, understanding that not all calories are created equal has ended my yo-yo dieting craze.

FOOD FOR THOUGHT

My early twenties were the lowest mental point in my life. I was chasing skinny and didn't care about my overall health. I would starve myself and restrict calories all through the week, then stay up late and party and binge eat on the weekends. I thought if I saved calories during the week, I wouldn't gain weight. I convinced myself that I would be healthy, happy, and worthy if I were skinny enough. To be honest, it worked for a while, and I finally got down to my goal weight, but I was miserable. I hated life. The number on the scale didn't fix my problems, and eventually, I gained the weight back.
This is a cycle that many of us are all too familiar with.

Calorie restriction is a sure-fire way to feel like a failure in the long run. Mechanisms within your body end up going into defense mode. This ultimately slows down metabolism and increases hunger.

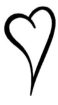

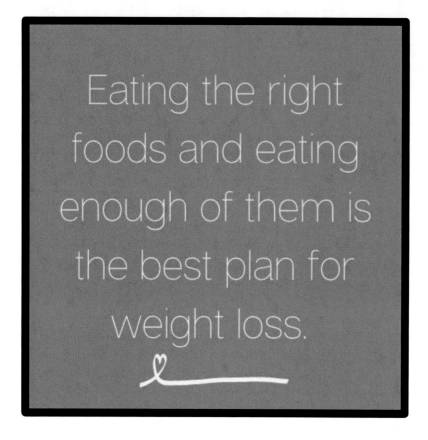

Eating the right foods and eating enough of them is the best plan for weight loss.

One of the most important tidbits of advice that I offer is this—stop looking for what you need to take out of your diet and start looking for what you can add to it. Crowd out unhealthy food with healthy choices!

GAINING CONTROL

When you gain control over what you eat and not how much you eat, the following will happen:

Gaining Control of Your Diet Leads To:

*Better Digestion

*Food Tastes Better

*Reduced Food Cravings

*Reduced Splurging

*Weight Loss

*Better Heart Health

*Controlled Blood Sugar

*A More Diverse Diet

I am frequently asked, "Are you vegan, vegetarian?" or "What diet are you on?"

I love veggies! But I also enjoy cheese and ice cream. I understand these foods don't nourish my body, so I don't eat them often.

Labeling my eating habits gives me anxiety. We have enough to stress about. I don't believe food should add to our worries.

BALANCE

Eating is a lifestyle for me. Ninety percent of the time, I consume whole food plant-based products, but if I'm craving cheese or ice cream, I eat that darn food.

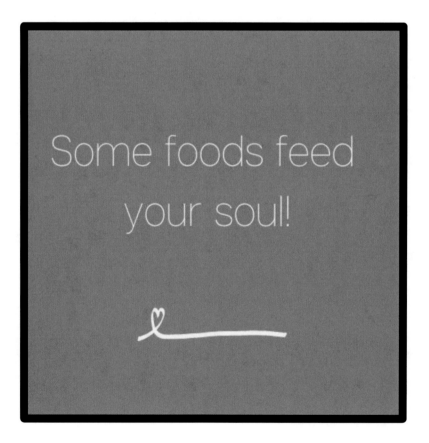

Some foods feed your soul!

The lesson in this? Balance is the key to mental and physical health. We can't work on one without working on the other.

I believe we are the experts of our bodies. I know what works for me based on how I feel. Therefore, I strive to help others learn what works for their **individual** make-up while keeping their optimal health at the forefront.

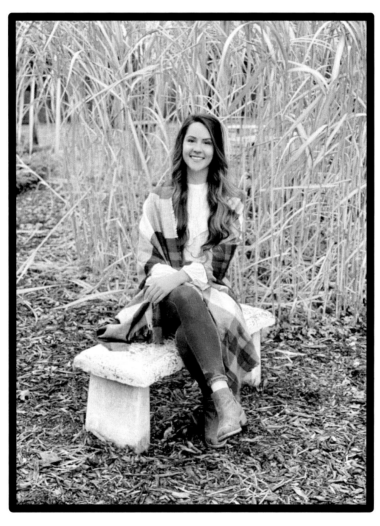

CHAPTER 5

HOW TO EAT MINDFULLY

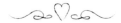

"If we could give every individual the right amount of nourishment and exercise, not too little and not too much, we would have found the safest way to health."- Hippocrates

I'm sure you are thinking, *This is great, Tia. So how do I eat more mindfully?*

START WITH SMALL CHANGES

*Eat slowly.
*Chew thoroughly.
*Eliminate distractions.
*Listen to physical hunger cues and stop eating as soon as you feel full.
*Learn to distinguish between true hunger and non-hunger triggers for eating.
*Engage your senses by noticing colors, smells, sounds, textures, and flavors.
*Learn to cope with guilt and anxiety about food.
*Eat to maintain overall health and well-being.
*Notice the effects food has on your feelings and mood.
*Be sure to appreciate your food.

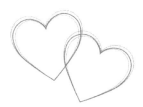

TRY IT OUT!

Take one meal and do the following: Start by asking yourself, *What am I hungry for and how hungry am I?* Then think, *How do these foods make me feel?* Picture your plate with bountiful, healthy foods that make you feel good. Prepare your plate, paying attention to the way it looks. Turn off the television and put your cell phone away. Eat slowly. *How does your food smell? How does it taste?* Roll it around on your tongue. Enjoy the sensual experience. Check-in often to ask yourself if you are full. Once you start to feel full—stop eating! Take a moment to be thankful for your meal.

SLOW DOWN!

If you choose to do one thing, eat slowly and chew your food!

Have you ever eaten so fast that you can't breathe after you're finished, and you end up feeling so full all you want to do is lie down? I confess that I have done this countless times.

Sometimes you end up eating far beyond the point of being sate. Sate means satisfying a desire or an appetite until full. Your body sends cues when you have eaten to satiety, but it can take up to twenty minutes to realize that you are full. So, if you eat quickly, your fullness signals may not arrive until you have already overeaten. This can cause binge eating.

> Slow down and make eating an intentional action instead of an automatic one.

When you learn to recognize the difference between physical hunger and fullness cues, you will be better able to distinguish between emotional triggers and true, physical hunger. You will become aware of the triggers that make you want to eat when you aren't hungry.

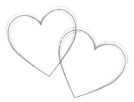

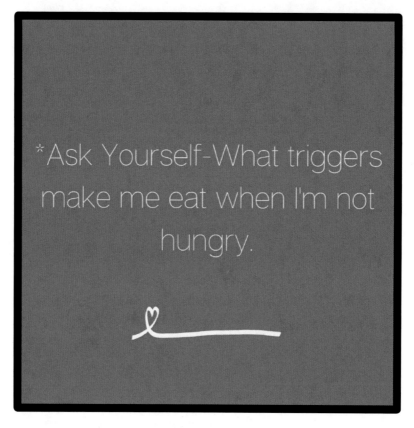

*Ask Yourself-What triggers make me eat when I'm not hungry.

Remember, you can go slowly, one meal at a time, and once you have the hang of it, you can expand mindful eating to all of your meals. Eventually, mindfulness will become more natural.

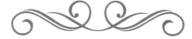

Five Tips for Eating Mindfully

1. Think about what you'd like to eat.

2. Think about how hungry you are.

3. Prepare a plate that reflects numbers one and two above.

4. Pay attention to the food – How it smells, how it feels in your mouth, how it tastes and whether you're enjoying it.

5. Pay attention to how full you are. *Stop Eating as soon as you feel full.

Are you ready to take the next steps?

Do overwhelming thoughts and emotions creep in when you think about living a healthier lifestyle?

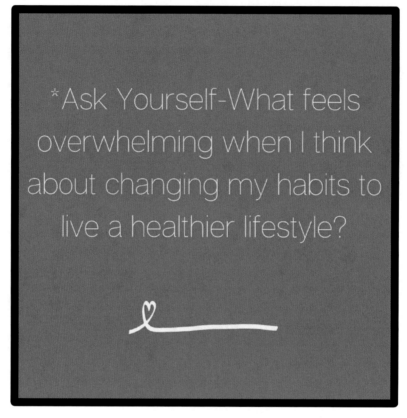

*Ask Yourself-What feels overwhelming when I think about changing my habits to live a healthier lifestyle?

Overwhelming thoughts and emotions are something I struggle with. They held me back from making the changes required to live the life I desired. Something that helped me move forward was the mantra, "Progress over perfection."

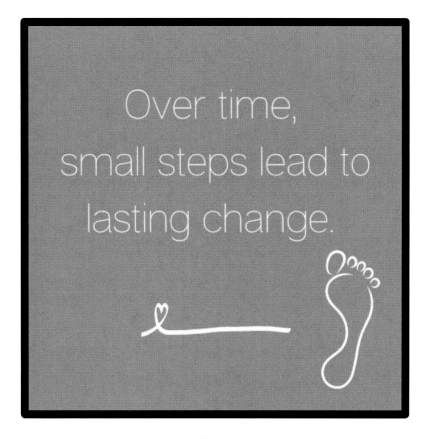

Health is a journey, not a destination. Small steps to health make the journey manageable and enjoyable! There is no reason to jump headfirst into making radical life changes. Start small and build on habits as you implement them successfully into your life.

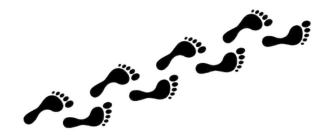

Here are small steps that you can implement. Try adding one at a time!

Small Steps That Go A Long Way

*Prioritize sleep: Schedule 7-9 hours each night. This is non-negotiable.

*Carry a water bottle: You're more likely to drink water when you have it on hand.

*Start with veggies: Plan your meals around veggies, and when going back for seconds, eat veggies first.

*Get moving: Start by walking 10 minutes a day, increasing slowly.

*Crowding out: Looking at what positive habits you can add to crowd out the habits you want to break.

*Grace: Giving yourself and others grace, knowing that change is not linear.

*Routine: When uncertainty hits, having a routine can help to stabilize you so that you can face the unknown.

*One step at a time: Small habits build up over time; no need to take on everything at once.

*Community: Leaning on others for support and accountability, especially on tough days.

KEEP A JOURNAL

A journal provides a method of self-discovery and it is habit changing. Most things in life worth having, typically do not fall on a linear path. One day you leap forward five steps and the next fall back three steps. On the days you fall back, you tend to have negative thought patterns spiraling in your mind. If you aren't aware of this, you will end up negatively fixating on the steps back. Even when in reality, you are still two steps ahead.

Keeping a journal of your journey can be helpful for many reasons. You can use your journals as a space to become aware of your inner monologue. You are able to bring awareness to the thoughts you have and intentionally choose the thoughts you want to have. It is evidence of what you have overcome and how far you have come. You can look back on your journals on the days you need a boost to keep moving. On the days you feel your best you can write an entry so you have something to look back on when you feel your worst. You can be your own voice of motivation when you read the words you personally wrote knowing good and bad days are inevitable.

Journaling can be what you make it. Try it out for a period of time so that you discover why keeping this practice in your life is rewarding and inspirational.

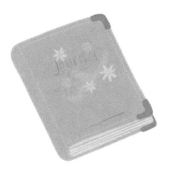

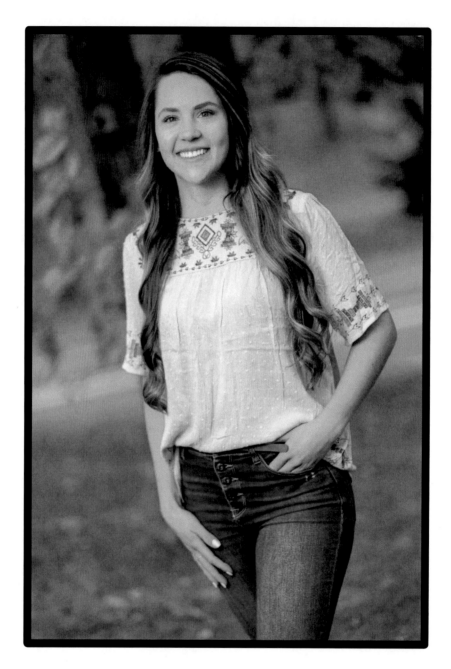

CHAPTER 6

EATING WHOLE FOODS

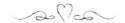

"Any food that requires enhancing by the use of chemical substances should in no way be considered a food."- John H. Tobe

When we were put on this earth, we were given everything we need to fuel our bodies, reproduce, evolve, and survive. It wasn't until the industrialization of food production that we started seeing a rise in cancers, obesity, and chronic disease. The good news is that humans have extraordinary powers to heal and thrive if put into the right environment.

THE IMPORTANCE OF WHOLE FOODS

Whole foods remain in their natural state and haven't been processed, packaged, or altered in any way. They contain all the minerals and vitamins that our bodies need, making them crucial for us.

Our bodies were not designed to digest the chemicals, preservatives, and things we can't even pronounce that have found their way into our food chain. Whether or not you have made the connection yet, I am sure that you have felt firsthand that processed foods make you feel lethargic, fatigued, and foggy-headed, while apples give a jolt of energy.

Let's examine other benefits of whole foods.

THE VIBRATIONAL ENERGY OF FOOD

I am not here to tell you to eat a certain way. My intention is to inform you how to make mindful choices aligned with your bio-individuality that help make you feel good.
I never considered how the food I ate impacted my vibrational energy because my focus was on how I looked externally. I didn't make the connection that my internal health influenced my external appearance until I started focusing on my mental health instead of being obsessed with chasing skinny.

I learned to be mindful about what types of energy I allowed into my life.

All things carry energy, including food, therefore, when eating, you consume energy. The type received varies based on what you eat. Mother Nature has gifted us with some of the purest nutrient-dense forms of energy needed to feel our best. However, when processing and manipulating whole foods, a heavy negative energy can result.

Pay attention to your energy levels before, during, and after you consume food. Our bio-individuality means we all can and will feel different after eating. We just need to listen to our body when it is communicating to us.

For the next week set your timer for ten minutes a day and keep a journal. Write down how you felt about your food choices today. Which foods made you feel good and gave you energy. What foods did you think you wanted and after you ate them you felt sluggish?

It is your choice. Do you want to soak up healthy vibrations or unnatural weighted down energy?

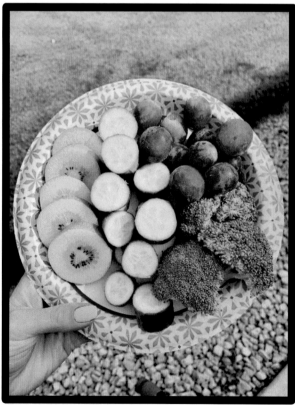

FIBER

Fiber does more than regulate bowel movements. It also reduces inflammation and the risk of cancer, diabetes, heart disease, obesity, and premature death.

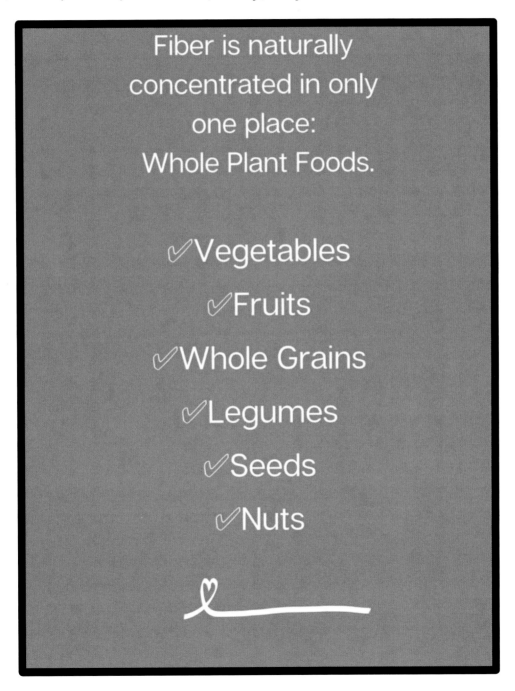

Fiber is naturally concentrated in only one place: Whole Plant Foods.

✓ Vegetables
✓ Fruits
✓ Whole Grains
✓ Legumes
✓ Seeds
✓ Nuts

Processed foods have significantly less fiber, and animal-derived foods have none. The goal is to crowd out processed foods by consuming more whole foods, which are a natural source of fiber. With this in mind, I still consume processed foods while being mindful of the label. Since label reading can become overwhelming, I stick to two main guidelines.

First, I review the ingredient list. Can I read everything listed? If I cannot understand the ingredients, it's likely my body won't recognize them either.
Second, Thanks to Dr. Greger, I now purchase my packaged foods by following the '5-to-1 rule.' This rule looks at the ratio of grams of carbohydrates to grams of dietary fiber.

You take the total grams of carbohydrates in a serving and divide them by the total grams of dietary fiber in a serving. The goal is to have it be 5 to 1 or less.
Example: See the Ezekiel 4:9 The Original Sprouted Grain Bread label below. First, I check the ingredients. Since I am able to read everything listed, it passes the first test. Second, I take the grams of carbs divided by grams of dietary fiber, 14/3=4.67. This is less than 5. It passes both tests, so I would purchase this packaged item.

Nutrition Facts

Serving Size 1 slice (34 g)
Serving Per Container 20

Amount Per Serving

Calories 80	Calories from Fat 5

	% Daily Values*
Total Fat 0.5g	1%
Saturated Fat 0g	0%
Trans Fat 0g	
Cholesterol 0mg	0%
Potassium 80mg	2%
Sodium 75mg	3%
Total Carbohydrate 14g	5%
Dietary Fiber 3g	12%
Sugars 0g	
Protein 4g	8%

Iron 4%	•	Thiamin 8%
Riboflavin 2%	•	Niacin 6%
Vitamin B6 4%	•	Folate 4%
Pantothenic Acid 2%	•	Phosphorus 8%
Magnesium 6%	•	Zinc 4%

*Percent Daily Values are based on a 2,000 calorie diet. Your Daily Values may be higher or lower depending on your calorie needs.

	Calories	2,000	2,500
Total Fat	Less than	65g	80g
Sat Fat	Less than	20g	25g
Cholesterol	Less than	300mg	300mg
Sodium	Less than	2400mg	2400mg
Total Carbohydrate		300g	375g
Dietary Fiber		25g	30g

Ezekiel 4:9
The Original Sprouted Grain Bread

Ingredients:

Organic Sprouted Wheat
Organic Sprouted Barley
Organic Sprouted Millet
Organic Sprouted Lentils
Organic Sprouted Soybeans
Spring Water
Organic Sprouted Spelt
Organic Honey
Organic Molasses
Organic Malted Barley
Yeast
Celtic Sea Salt®.

Certified Organic by the Washington State Dept. of Agriculture (Olympia, WA 98504)

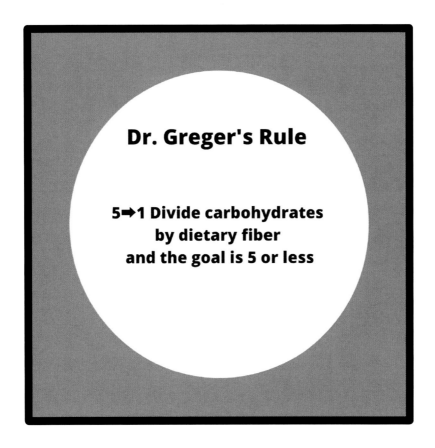

Dr. Greger's Rule

**5➡1 Divide carbohydrates
by dietary fiber
and the goal is 5 or less**

ORGANIC? YES OR NO?

Even though I knew that pesticides and chemicals were unhealthy, I still wasn't sure if it was worth buying organic produce.

It is thought that organic produce is more health-promoting. The antioxidant phytonutrient content in organic produce is higher. Phytonutrients are how plants defend themselves in their environment. The fact is, the greater the stress level on plants while growing, the more phytonutrients they manufacture. Phytonutrients are antistress agents for plants. When we consume these antistress agents, they work as messengers in our bodies to increase our physiological resilience. In turn, food plays a role in modifying the expression of our genes related to overall health.

I believe the benefits of consuming non-organic produce far outweigh the risks of pesticides. However, my conclusion is that, organic or not, choose to eat more whole foods. Pick up fruits and vegetables at the store, grow your own, or shop at your local farmer's market.

Let me take a moment to climb onto my soapbox.

Use your consumer buying power to tell the food industries that we value the health of our bodies and the planet. Cut back on processed food in environmentally unfriendly packaging. When possible, eliminate those pesticides and chemicals.

Things won't change until our purchase habits change.

Money Talks!

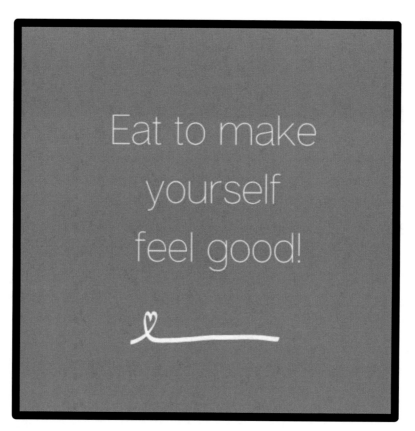

POWER FOODS

Power foods provide optimal health benefits and contain the richest amount of nutrients for the least amount of calories. I truly believe all whole foods are power foods but below are a few of my favorites.

Dark leafy greens: Nutrient-dense foods such as dark leafy greens have many benefits, from strengthening our immune systems to mood-boosting superpowers. They are packed full of magnesium, calcium, iron, zinc, potassium, and vitamins A, C, E, and K.

Cruciferous vegetables: Broccoli, cauliflower, brussel sprouts, bok choy, kale, cabbage, kohlrabi, radishes, and turnips, are just a few cruciferous plants. These vegetables contain antioxidants, fiber, calcium, and vitamins A, C, and K. They are cancer-fighting, inflammation-reducing, immune-boosting, toxin reducers that promote healing within the body.

Avocados: Avocados are a magical fruit (yes, technically a fruit) packed full of macronutrients and micronutrients that our bodies require to thrive. They are a healthy source of fat that contains tryptophan, folate, omega-3 fatty acids, pantothenic acid, vitamin E, and vitamin B6.

Berries: Berries are bursting with antioxidants, phytonutrients, and fiber. They also contain the numerous vitamins and minerals that we need for optimal health. Berries are naturally low in fat and calories, promoting healthy weight, energy, and vitality.

Chia seeds: These tiny seeds are gentle detoxing, energy-boosting, fatigue, and inflammation-fighting powerhouses. They provide an abundance of vitamins and minerals, as well as being a source of protein, fiber, and omega 3 and 6 fatty acids. They are also high in antioxidants. An added bonus is they help you feel full longer.
Whole foods, in general, are the way to go. They contain vitamins, minerals, antioxidants, phytonutrients, and many other things that our bodies require for optimal health and a thriving lifestyle. Ideally, we should consume a variety of whole foods daily. Challenge yourself and aim to see how many foods in a day you can eat that aren't processed. Then try to outdo the previous day's total.

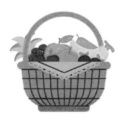

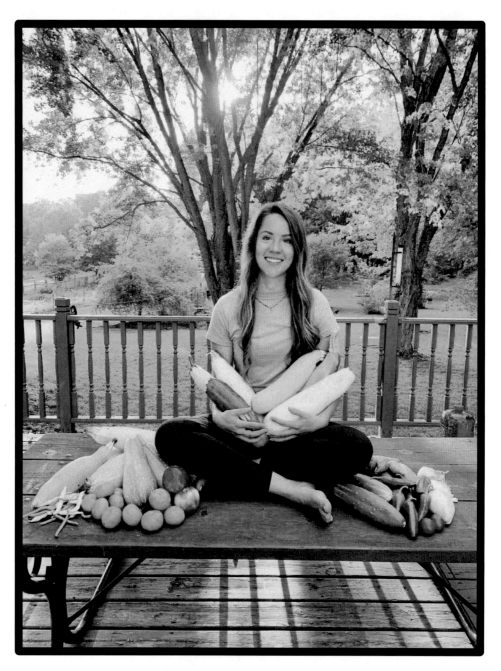

CHAPTER 7

PRIMARY FOODS

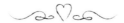

"To keep the body in good health is a duty, otherwise we shall not be able to keep our mind strong and clear."-Buddha.

The IIN curriculum opened my eyes to the depth behind health and food choices. Wellness goes far beyond the food we eat. We need food to survive, but primary food goes deeper than this and emphasizes that we are multidimensional beings. It encourages us to look at our health from a big-picture perspective.

PRIMARY FOODS

Primary Foods are more than what is on your plate. Healthy relationships, regular physical activity, a fulfilling career, and a spiritual practice can fill your soul and satisfy your hunger for life. They also affect what you choose to eat. If you lack in one of the twelve life areas, you are more inclined to eat things that don't make you feel well. For example, if you are in a negative relationship or hate your job, you are more inclined to eat unhealthy food **to fill that void.**

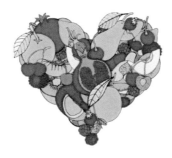

Primary Foods

Primary food brings awareness to the full picture of well-being through the 12 areas that make up the Circle of Life:

Joy

Spirituality

Creativity

Finances

Career

Home environment

Home cooking

Physical activity

Health

Education

Social life

Relationships

Primary foods are what nourishes us off the plate, and secondary food is the food we eat. They need to be examined together in relation to one another.

Primary foods are connected to secondary food cravings. We tend to make food choices for many reasons other than hunger. See the chart below to view the areas that affect our food choices.

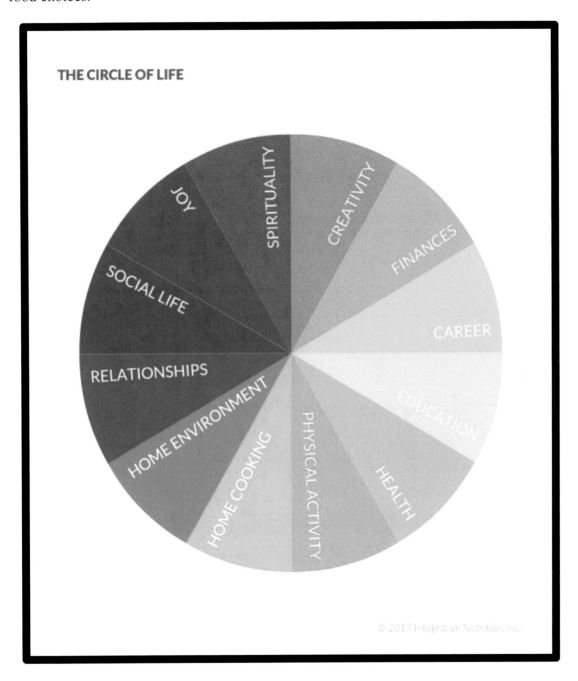

THE CIRCLE OF LIFE

SPIRITUALITY
CREATIVITY
JOY
FINANCES
SOCIAL LIFE
CAREER
RELATIONSHIPS
EDUCATION
HOME ENVIRONMENT
HOME COOKING
PHYSICAL ACTIVITY
HEALTH

© 2017 Integrative Nutrition, Inc.

Evaluating the areas of primary food allows you to identify where imbalances exist in your current season of life. When you take a step back and look at your life as a whole, you can find the root cause—not just the symptom—of the how, what and why of what you eat. Aim to be curious about your behaviors and habits around food, without being judgmental. This allows you to evaluate your choices and habits from a heart-centered approach. Curiosity will help you to develop self-compassion and self-awareness. When evaluating your circle of life do the following:

1. Within each area place a dot on the line to indicate your level of satisfaction. The center of the circle represents dissatisfaction and outside satisfaction. Most people will fall somewhere in between and that is okay.

2. Connect the dots you place on each line to see your Circle of Life.

3. Identify the imbalances you see and determine where to focus more time and energy to bring balance into your life.

Example:

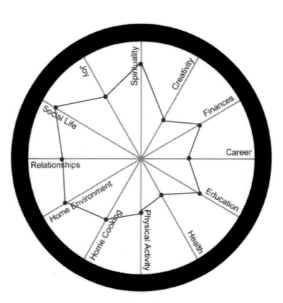

This isn't a one-and-done check-the-box kind of deal. These areas need to be evaluated often. Do honest check-ins when you feel an imbalance to see which area(s) need a little extra attention.

I hope this tool helps you to identify imbalances. It can and should be used often since satisfaction in these areas shifts in every season of life. And remember, when Primary Food is balanced and satiating, your life feeds you, making what you eat secondary.

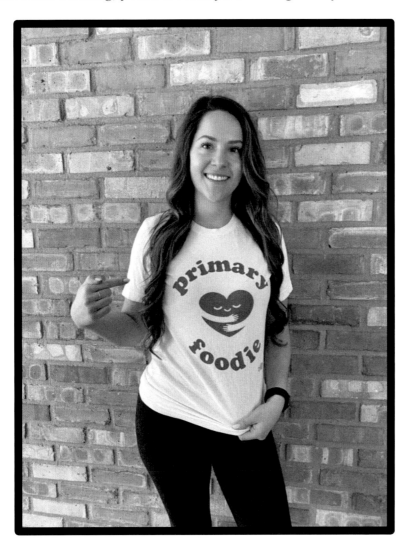

CHAPTER 8

EATING FOR HAPPINESS

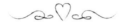

"One cannot think well, love well, sleep well if one has not dined well." - Virginia Woolf

The great news is that by changing what and how you eat, you can positively influence your mood and strengthen your health at the same time.

FOOD AND MOOD

Our bodies compensate for highly processed foods by downregulating dopamine levels. Our bodies reduce our pleasure and feel-good hormones when we eat highly processed foods. This realization changed my life and made the pieces of my mental health journey make sense. Of course, I feel foggy-brained and fatigued when I don't eat to nourish my body. It is empowering to know that my mental and emotional health is directly affected by what I eat and that I have control over this.

On some level, many of us understand that highly processed foods affect our bodies physically, but we don't take the time to consider its mental and emotional aspects. What can we do to fix this?

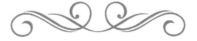

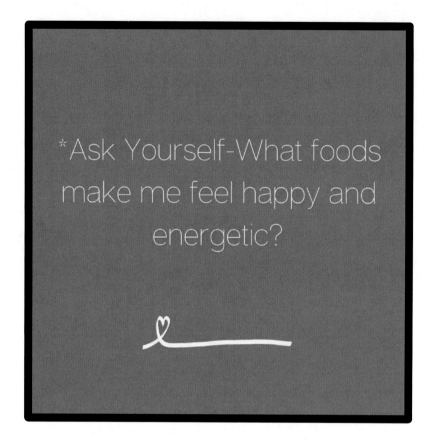

*Ask Yourself-What foods make me feel happy and energetic?

Remember, when you learn to listen to your body, it will tell you what it needs.

Eating to Feel Good

*Keep It Whole

*Cook At Home

*Limit Refined Carbs

*Limit Processed Food

*Create Structure

*Balance Your Plate

Let's examine the tips from above.

1. Keep it whole. Aim to consume whole foods. Whole foods are those that are found in nature. They don't typically require flashy packaging.

2. Experiment with cooking at home. (I have included a chapter of delicious recipes and food templates that you can try.) Cooking for yourself is almost guaranteed to be more nutritious. It is difficult to know the quality of ingredients used in restaurant settings.

3. Limit refined carbohydrates and foods made from white sugar.

4. Limit processed food and foods with fancy packaging.

5. Create Structure. Plan mealtime to maintain consistent eating times. Avoid skipping meals. This helps to regulate hormones and keep your blood sugar stable. Have an idea of what you are going to eat, prior to feeling hungry.

6. Balance your plate. Aim to consume quality proteins, carbohydrates, and fats at every meal. Strive for at least half your meal to be vegetables.

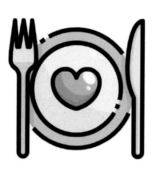

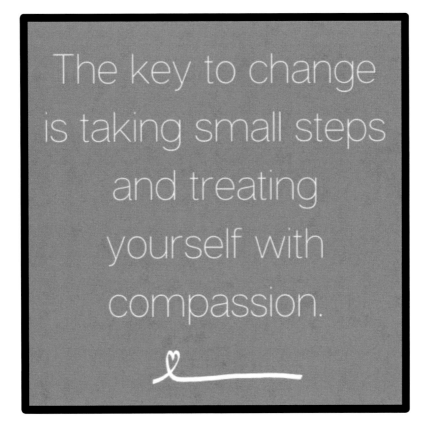

I can't say it enough, making small changes and treating yourself with compassion will lead to a happier, healthier life.

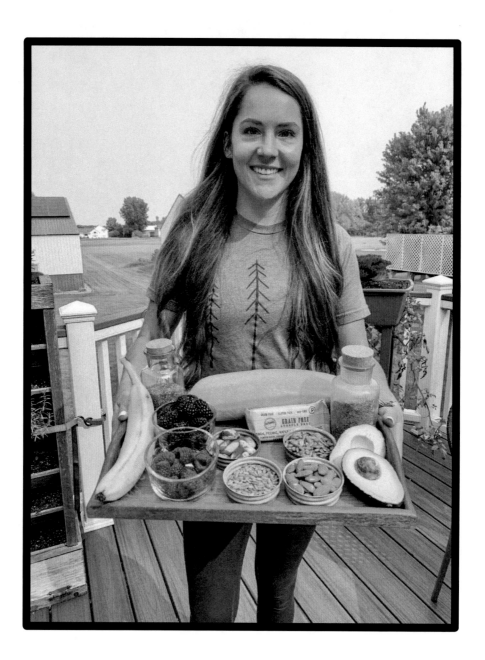

CHAPTER 9

TREATING YOURSELF WITH KINDNESS AND COMPASSION

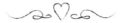

"Talk to yourself like you would to someone you love."- Brene Brown

Do you eat as if you love yourself? This is a critical part of being healthy.

LOVE YOURSELF

Think about what you ate this morning. Did you feed yourself a glorious abundance of colorful food? Or did you just pile some pre-packaged, processed convenience food into that gorgeous mouth of yours? Take a deep dive and understand that every molecule of food that you put into your body directly affects your energy, your vibrance, your skin—your everything! It all starts with you.

Take care of yourself today so that you can be stronger tomorrow.

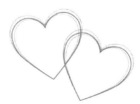

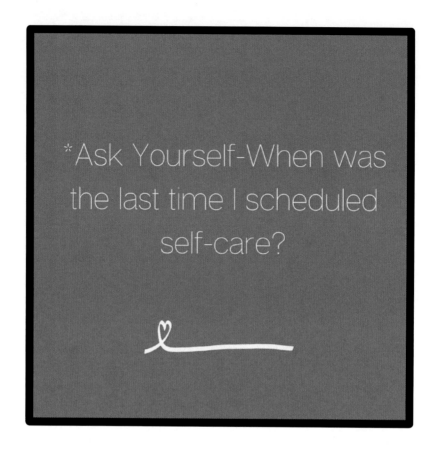

*Ask Yourself-When was the last time I scheduled self-care?

SELF-CARE

The importance of self-care is underestimated by many. Excuses flood our minds about why we can't take time to practice self-care. *I don't have time. I have to be everything for everyone. Self-care is selfish. I can't put myself first. It's not a big deal. It doesn't truly make a difference in my health.*

However, health effects compound over time.

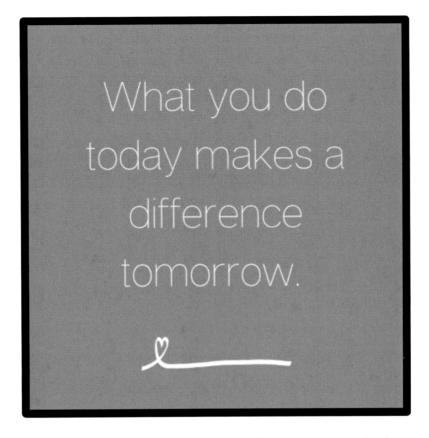

You would never expect your electronics to work if the battery was dead or your car to run if it was out of gas. Do you expect your body to function day after day without properly recharging or refueling it?

Self-care doesn't have to be elaborate, expensive, or time-consuming. It is individualized to what makes you feel recharged.

Here are some basic things that you can do to take care of your beautiful body.

Self-Care Basics

*Stay Hydrated

*Eat Food That Fuels Your Body

*Get Outside

*Move Your Body Daily

*Sleep

Since I have already addressed the importance of eating healthy foods that make you feel happy, energetic, and satiated, I will take some time to talk about the importance of hydration, getting outside, staying active, and adequate sleep.

STAY HYDRATED

I'm all about the "what can I add to my diet" mindset. The easiest place to start was water and making sure I was consciously consuming enough daily to remain hydrated. We all know we should drink water, yet seventy-five percent of Americans are chronically dehydrated.

For optimal health, aim for half your body weight in ounces daily! **Start slowly and work your way up. Begin with one glass of water at a time.**

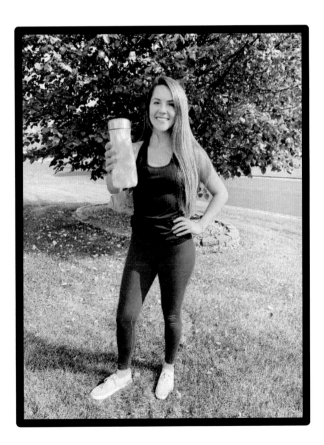

GET OUTSIDE

Our health goes beyond the food we consume. We can eat all of the right foods and still lack in many areas if we aren't spending our days feeding our souls. It's scientifically proven that we need time in nature. Ecotherapy refers to the various physical and psychological benefits of being outside.

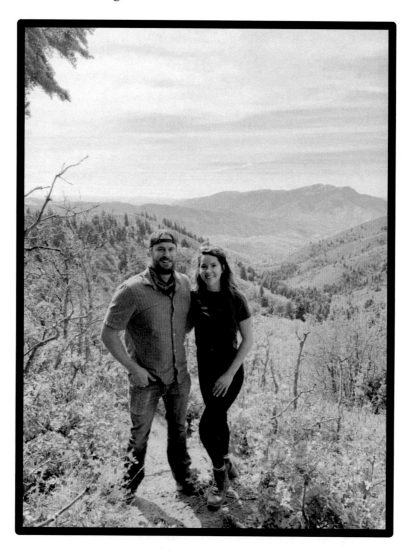

Spending time in nature, in solitude, or with those you love improves your quality of life!

Get Outside!

*Eases Depression and Anxiety

*Improves Focus

*Strengthens Immunity

*Lowers Cortisol Levels, Heart Disease, and Blood Pressure

*Improves Sleep

*Overall Happier, Healthier Lifestyle

EXERCISE

For many people, exercise comes from wanting to burn a lot of calories, which doesn't necessarily serve our bodies. I recommend finding activities that make you feel good. My go-to's are yoga and walking. I add in strength training when my body says I need it.

Whatever I choose to do, I listen to my body, and I don't strain or harm it in any way. One of my favorite things is to get outside and spend time with Mother Nature. I recommend that you also choose movements that make you love and appreciate your body!

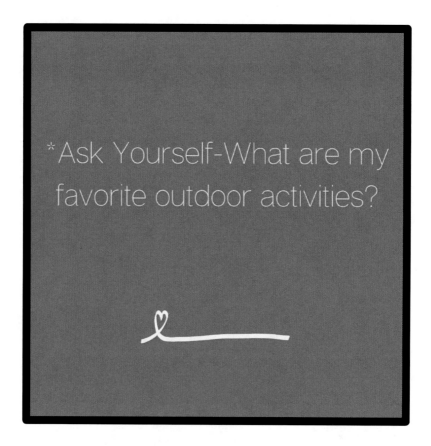

SLEEP

Do not undervalue sleep. Proper rest is mandatory for stress management, maintaining a healthy weight, and overall health.

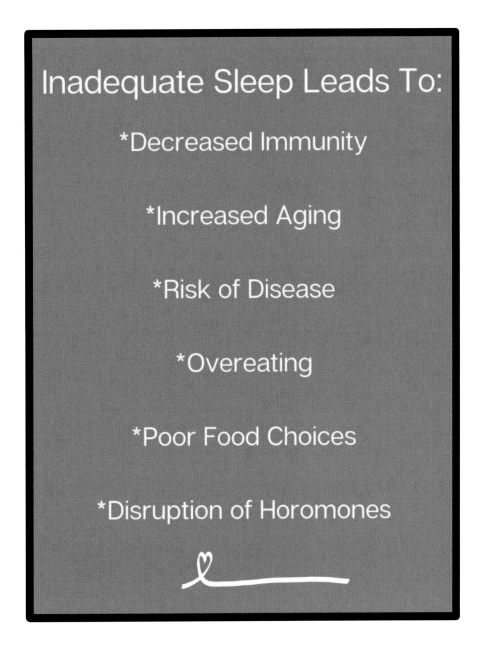

If you are currently getting less than six hours of sleep, start by going to bed five minutes earlier and adding five minutes each night until you are up to at least seven hours. Pay attention to how you feel in the morning, then improve your sleep to fit your needs. Your body knows what is best and will insist on what it needs if you are willing to listen. Here are some more tips to help you:

Improving Sleep

*Prioritize it. View it as an act of self-care.

*Form a night-time routine.

*Limit screen time such as television and phone right before bed.

*Schedule 7-9 hours of sleep.

*Avoid harsh lighting an hour before you go to sleep.

*Avoid eating before bed.

*Do yoga or meditate before bed.

FIND WHAT WORKS FOR YOU

In the end, self-care will look different for each individual. For you, it might be that yoga class you have always wanted to take, a night out with the girls, reading a book while taking a bath, listening to your favorite music, or petting your puppy. Whatever it is, be sure to make that regular date with yourself.

I will leave you with one final thought about self-care:

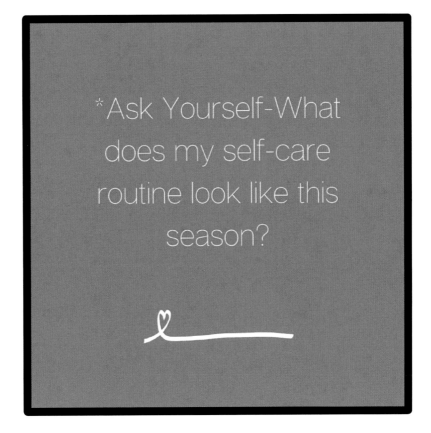
*Ask Yourself-What does my self-care routine look like this season?

CHAPTER 10

THE IMPORTANCE OF KINDNESS

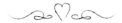

"A single act of kindness throws out roots in all directions, and the roots spring up and make new trees. The greatest work that kindness does to others is that it makes them kind to themselves." -Frederick William Faber.

We tend to judge ourselves based on our intentions and judge others based on their actions. Is it fair? Not really, but it's reality. We can have the best intentions in the world, but no one can see them. So, give others the benefit of the doubt. You never really know what their intentions were or what's going on in their life. Be the start of the ripple effect of kindness.

BE KIND AND BRAVE

Kindness is food for the body and mind. It increases self-esteem, empathy, compassion, and connection to others. It boosts serotonin and dopamine levels and allows the brain to release endorphins, improving mood. And don't forget the most crucial par

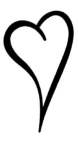

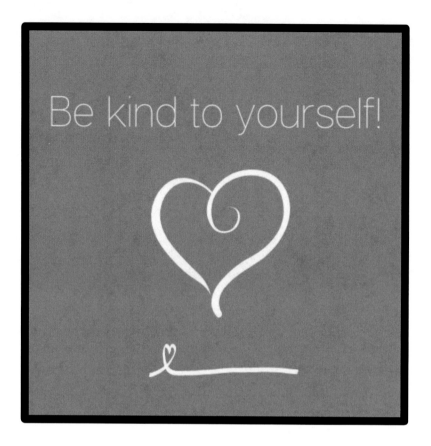

POSITIVE AFFIRMATIONS:

I am a firm believer in shifting intentions into affirmations and living them out as if they are already true.

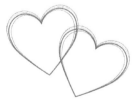

> Showering kindness on yourself and others is one of the most important things you can do for your health. ♡

Here are some affirmations that I have used in the past:

*I live in the now with complete acceptance.

*My mood is up to me, and I choose for it to be joyful.

*Every decision I make creates more abundance in my life.

*Everything in my life is working out for the best and highest possible good for all.

*I fully trust in divine timing.

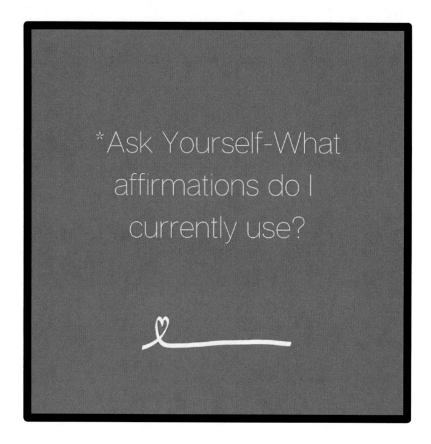

*Ask Yourself-What affirmations do I currently use?

We will come back to affirmations later in this book, and I will challenge you to create positive statements.

BEING INTENTIONAL

Like all personal values, deciding to be kind is a decision we consciously make, then must maintain daily. By intentionally being kind to those around us, we positively impact our internal thoughts. We are able to be kind to ourselves and make decisions from a heart-centered mindset that leads to decisions we are proud of. This includes our food choices. We tend to make decisions based on how we feel about ourselves at that moment. When we are feeling positively about ourselves, we are going to choose foods that reflect this.

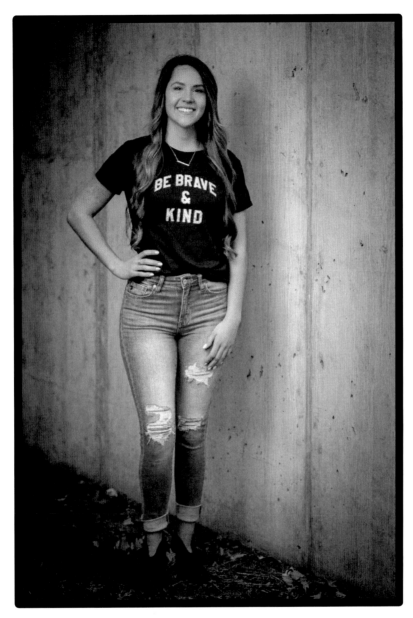

CHAPTER 11
WRAP-UP

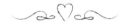

"Be the change that you wish to see in the world." - **Mahatma Gandhi**

The more we pay attention to our lifestyle and eating habits, the more we can identify connections between how we live and how we feel. If we don't have awareness, we will never see what needs to change.

Change is not the enemy; resisting change is where the pain lies. Therefore, embrace where you are today and invest in where you want to be tomorrow.

In today's world, it is more important than ever to:

✓ Pay attention to our health

✓ Invest in our health

✓ Take responsibility for our health

Remember, your health is in your hands, so stop waiting for external circumstances to initiate change within.

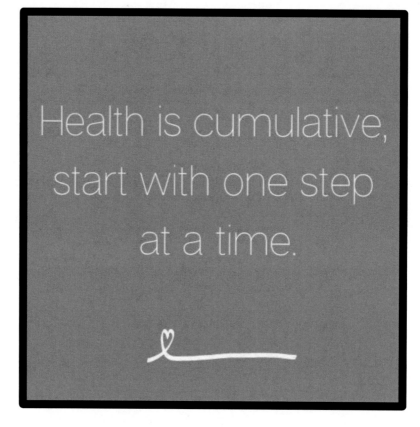

Finally, remember that food should be an enjoyable part of your life and not another stressor. Have fun experimenting with food to find what works for your body. Give yourself grace as you navigate your journey. Eating mindfully doesn't happen overnight. Some days we fall short, and that's okay.

POST ASSESSMENT

It is time to pull out the assessment you took before beginning this book. Complete it again to see if your answers have changed. Evaluate yourself and ask *Where have I made progress? Where do I need to focus my energy?* Revisit these questions as often as needed.

Self Assessment

Where do you fall with these statements? Where do you want to fall with them? How can you start to implement mindful eating habits into your life?

1. I take the time to notice how hungry I am before I start eating to make the appropriate food choices and control the portion size?

2. I eat my meals while watching TV, scrolling social media, listening to audio, reading emails, text, or making calls?

3. I eat to the point of being uncomfortable? I often want to do 'nothing' after I eat?

4. I eat so quickly I barely taste the food, notice the texture, think about the appearance or appreciate how it got on my plate?

5. I find myself staring into the refrigerator/pantry for reasons other than being hungry?

Self Assessment
Page 2

6. When I notice my attention drifting during meals, I refocus my thoughts back to the eating experience?

7. When I feel hungry my first instinct is to avoid the feeling and distract myself so I don't eat?

8. I always finish my plate, even when I know I am full before all the food is gone?

9. I make food choices based on the quality and quantity of what those around me eat?

10. I accept my body as is at all times without judgment?

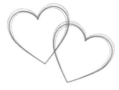

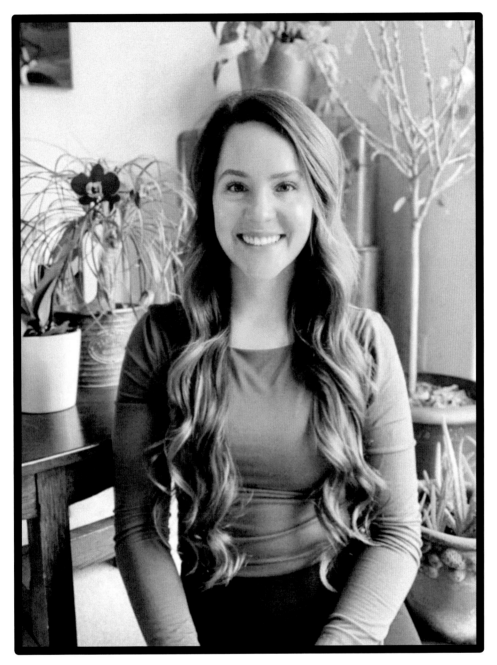

CHAPTER 12

IN THE KITCHEN

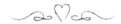

"You don't have to cook fancy or complicated masterpieces—just good food from fresh ingredients"- Julie Child

Here are some of my favorite go-to recipes to get you started on your heart-centered approach to nourishing your body.

Green Smoothie

Ingredients: add fruit, raw honey, or pure maple syrup to sweeten to taste

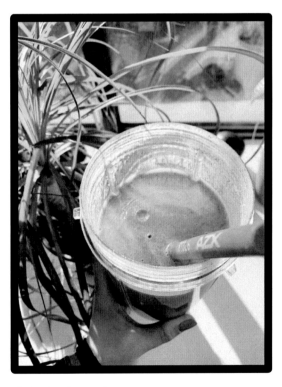

- 1-2 handfuls of leafy greens
- ½ avocado
- 8-12 oz. of plant milk or water
- 7 ice cubes
- 2 tablespoons of flaxseeds
- 2 Tablespoons of chia seeds
- 1 teaspoon of cinnamon
- 1 teaspoon of turmeric (or turmeric root)
- 1 teaspoon of ginger (or ginger root)
- 1 scoop plant-based protein vanilla *optional

Procedure
1. Combine all ingredients in a blender until desired consistency.
2. Enjoy your creamy smoothie.

Veggie Pasta Salad

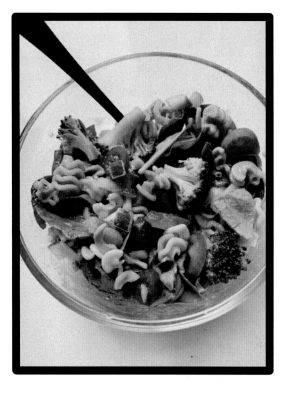

Ingredients:

(Any veggies can be added or subtracted to please your taste. Amounts can be altered depending on how much you want to make as well. Can't go wrong here!)

- 1 box of Banza Rotini made from chickpeas (or desired pasta alternative)
- 1 cup of Italian dressing
- ½ cup of onions chopped
- 1 cup of bell peppers chopped
- 1 fresh jalapeno chopped
- ½ cup broccoli chopped
- ½ cup radishes chopped
- ½ cup cucumber chopped
- ½ cup diced tomatoes or small cherry tomatoes
- ½ cup cauliflower chopped

Procedure:
1. Cook pasta by following the instructions on the box.
2. Chop desired veggies.
3. Mix cooked pasta, chopped veggies (raw), and dressing in a big mixing bowl. (If you desire more dressing, add to taste)
4. Let the mixture sit in the fridge for 30 minutes minimum. Add fresh spinach right before eating.

Pasta and Veggies

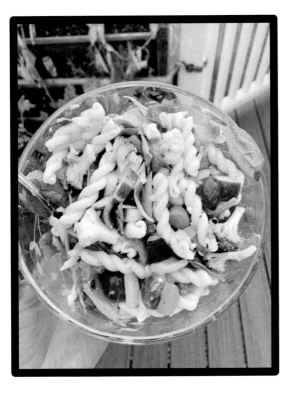

Ingredients:

(Any veggies can be added or subtracted to please your taste. Amounts can be altered depending on how much you want to make as well. Can't go wrong here!)

- 1 box of Banza Rotini made from chickpeas (or desired pasta alternative)
- ½ cup basil pesto
- ½ cup alfredo
- ½ cup of onions chopped
- 1 cup of bell peppers chopped
- 1 fresh jalapeno chopped
- 1 cup chopped Brussel sprouts
- ½ cup broccoli chopped
- ½ cup radishes chopped
- ½ cup cauliflower chopped
- ¼ cup chopped mushrooms

Procedure:
1. Cook the pasta by following the instructions on the box.
2. Chop desired veggies.
3. Sauté veggies in 2-4 Tablespoons of water for 10 minutes, or to desired texture.
4. Mix cooked pasta, sautéed veggies, and desired sauce in a pan. Let the combination warm for 5 minutes until one temperature.

"Stuffed' Recipe

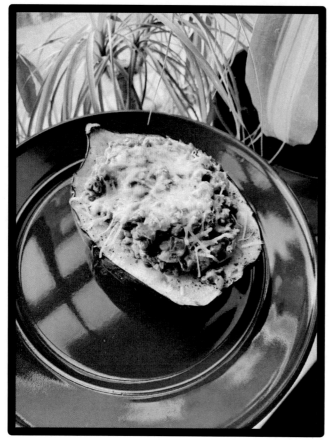

Great for stuffing mushrooms, bell peppers, jalapenos, tomatoes, and more!

Any veggies can be added or subtracted to please your taste

Ingredients: (*dairy-free alternatives can be used*)

- ¼ brick of cream cheese
- ¼ cup fresh blue cheese crumbles
- ½ cup onions chopped
- 1 cup bell peppers chopped
- 1 fresh jalapeno chopped
- ¼ cup mushrooms chopped
- 1 cup cooked quinoa
- ½ pound spicy sausage *optional
- ¼ teaspoon of oregano
- ¼ teaspoon of chili powder
- ¼ teaspoon of garlic
- pepper to taste

Procedure:
1. Cook quinoa by following the instructions on the box.
2. Brown spicy sausage if using meat.
3. Chop desired veggies into small bits and sauté for 10 minutes in 2-4 Tablespoons of water.
4. Lower heat to simmer. Combine veggies and quinoa (add meat if using), melt in the cream cheese, and blue cheese crumbles.
5. Stir in spices.
6. Stuffed mushroom caps, bell peppers, jalapenos, or desired stuffable vegetables. Bake in the oven at 400 degrees for 10-15 minutes or in an air fryer for 8 minutes.

Zucchini Lasagna

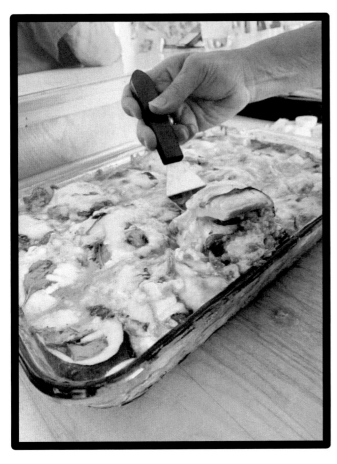

Ingredients:

- 3 zucchinis thinly sliced (the best you can)
- 1 pound ground spicy sausage/beef/turkey (*spice level to taste, also great meatless*)
- 1 sautéed white onion
- ½ jar of marinara sauce
- 16 ounces cottage cheese
- 12 ounces mozzarella cheese
- spinach
- mushrooms
- jalapenos *optional
- 1 egg
- ⅛ teaspoon pepper
- ½ teaspoon dry parsley

Procedure:
1. Mix the cottage cheese, mozzarella, egg, pepper, and parsley
2. Mix the meat, marinara, and onion
3. *Zucchini is over 90% water. To keep your dish from becoming a watery mess, roast the slices at 450°F for 12 minutes. Then cook the lasagna and let cool for 15 to 20 minutes before cutting.
4. Layer in a glass pan
   *Meat sauce
   *Zucchini
   *Cheese mix
   *Spinach
   *Mushrooms
   *Jalapenos
   *Meat sauce

*Zucchini
*Cheese mix
*Spinach
*Top off with more mozzarella
5. Bake in the oven at 375°F for 40 minutes or until the top starts to golden.

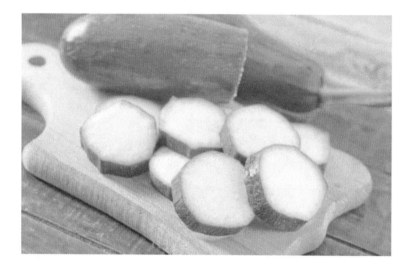

Whole Meal Salad Outline

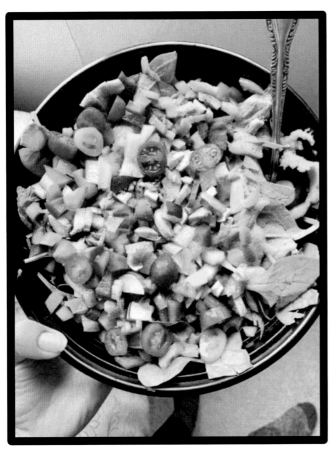

1. Choose a leafy green
-Spinach, kale, lettuce, baby greens, leafy green mix, arugula, watercress, etc.
-Roughly one handful or 1 cup per person

2. Choose a bean/legume
-Chickpeas, navy beans, black beans, edamame, kidney beans, green peas, lentils, etc.
-Roughly ½ to 1 cup of legumes per person

3. Choose vegetables
- Choose vegetables that appeal to you in their raw forms.
-Use ½ to 1 whole vegetable of each kind you choose

4. Add raw nuts or seeds
-optional. Any raw nuts or seeds of your liking, 2 tablespoons or a small handful per person

5. Season/dress the salad
-Add any fresh or dried herbs and/or spices: cumin, black pepper, cayenne pepper, oregano, basil, garlic, ginger, etc.
-Desired dressings: balsamic, vinegar, apple cider, lemon or lime juice, etc.

Whole Meal Template

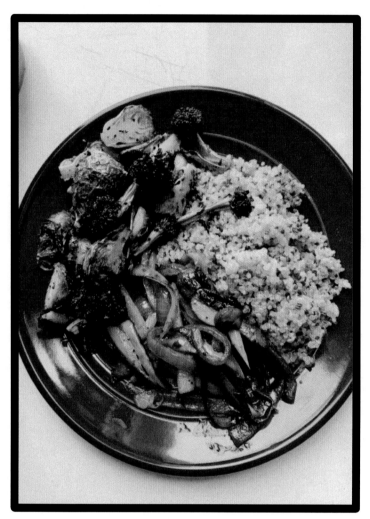

1. Choose a starchy vegetable or a grain.
   -Starchy vegetables: potatoes, sweet potatoes, cassava, or winter squash
   -Grains: whole rice, quinoa, buckwheat, millet, amaranth, or sorghum

2. Choose desired vegetables
   -Choose veggies ideal in cooked forms like broccoli, cauliflower, asparagus, Brussel sprouts, eggplant, zucchini, onions, carrots, etc.

3. Choose a legume if desired.
   -Beans, bean sprouts, tofu, tempeh

4. Add seasoning/sauce
   -Seasonings: fresh herbs and spices
   -Sauce: creamy nut/seed sauce, balsamic vinegar, puree, citrus juice, etc.

CHAPTER 13

RESOURCES

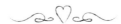

"Each patient carries his own doctor inside him." - Norman Cousins

Tools to help you on your Journey

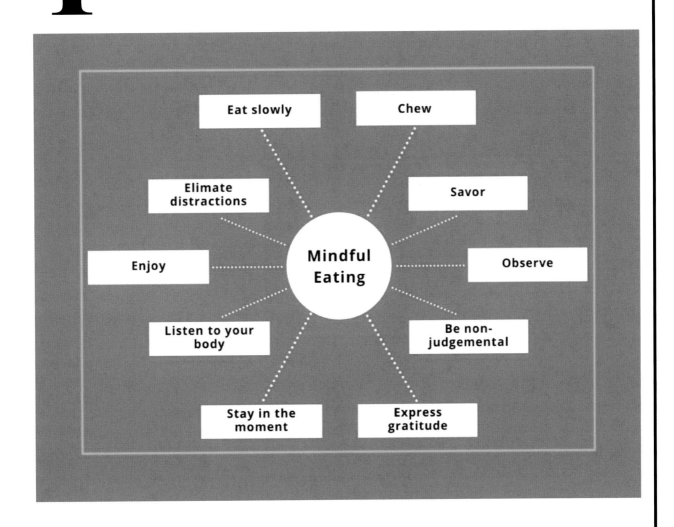

Tips For Holiday Eating

*We can enjoy holidays and all they have to offer by honoring our hunger and respecting our fullness.

*One unhealthy meal does not make you unhealthy.

*We do not need to earn our food by overexercising or depriving ourselves beforehand.

*You won't remember the calories you consumed at your family meal, you will remember the memories you created.

*We are permitted to challenge the assumption that overindulgence is a foregone conclusion of the season. Constant overeating on holidays doesn't have to be your truth.

Keystone Habits

Invest in YOURSELF .

Investing in yourself doesn't have to be hard, you don't need to over complicate it, or change everything you're currently doing. Making this investment has been manageable for me through the use of Keystone Habits.
.

What are Keystone Habits?
Small changes or habits that people introduce into their routines that unintentionally carry over into other aspects of their lives.

.

My Keystone Habits:
* 8 hours of sleep
* making my bed every morning
* Vegetables at every meal
* Intentionally moving my body for 30 minutes a day
* Gratitude/journaling

Ask Yourself- What are my Keystone Habits?

Creating Affirmations

The affirmations that I choose for myself are intentional. Here are some that have helped me:

*I know I can handle anything that comes my way.
*I give myself permission to feel joy without guilt.
*I am strong enough to challenge my beliefs and choose ones that align with my soul.
*I am free to feel how I want to feel.
*I am allowed to take time to get my heart and mind in sync.

Tips for writing your affirmations:

1. Express in the present tense. Ex. I will... I can... I know...
2. Make them positive.
3. Chose ones that are "right" for you.
4. Create the sense that you believe they are true.
5. Make them specific.

Write your affirmations on a fancy notecard, and keep them where you will see them. Tack them on your refrigerator, your bathroom mirror, on your nightstand, or your cell phone. The important thing is to find the method that works for you. I recommend re-evaluating them on a regular basis. I rethink mine at the beginning of each month.

What affirmations do you choose? Have fun!

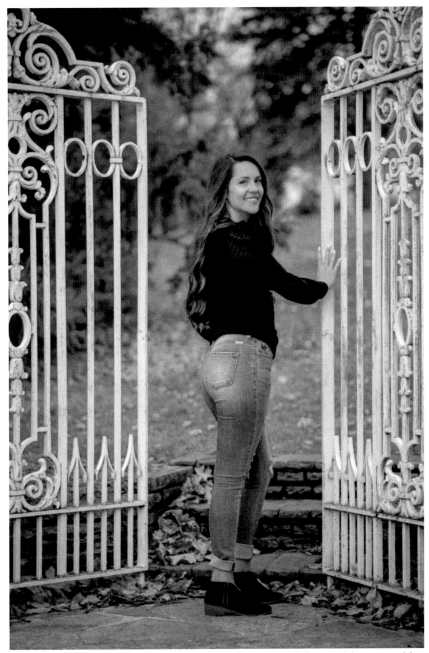

To learn more about Tia: https://www.crownandcompasslifecoaching.com/tia-s-tips
You can contact Tia at: tia@crownandcompasscoaching.com and on Instagram at
tia.morell

Made in the USA
Middletown, DE
06 June 2021

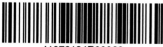

41076134R00060